NUTRITION DURING PREGNANCY:

Staying healthy, fit and comfortable.

MELANIE

MELANIE

Copyright © 2012 Author Name

All rights reserved.

ISBN: 9781521527283

CONTENTS

Introduction 6

Chapter 1:

7 golden rules of nutrition for pregnant women 8

Rule 1 – don't eat for two 8

Rule 2 – getting enough folic acid 9

Rule 3 – getting adequate iron 10

Rule 4 – getting enough zinc 11

Rule 5 – boosting calcium intake 12

Rule 6 – focusing on fiber 14

Rule 7 – avoiding harmful foods and drinks 15

Chapter 2:

Things to consider in the first trimester of pregnancy 17

Dealing with morning sickness 17

Certain nutrient-deficiency is linked to miscarriage 20

Foods are high in folic acid 21
1. Dark leafy green 21
2. Bean, peas and lentils 21
3. Avocados 22
4. Cauliflower and broccoli 22
5. Seeds and nuts 22

Chapter 3: Nutritional requirements
in the second trimester of pregnancy 23
Protein 23
Omega-3 fatty acids 25

Chapter 4: Staying healthy and safe
in the last trimester of pregnancy 28
How to manage healthy weight in the last trimester of pregnancy 28
How many calories do you need during pregnancy? 30
Tips to manage your weight: 31
1. Eat moderately and often 31
2. Drink enough water 32
3. Choosing nonfat dairy products and skimmed milk 32
4. Reducing junk foods 32
5. Eliminating sugar and sweetened drinks 33
6. Don't skip your breakfast 33
7. Eating more fruits and vegetables 33
The importance of iron sufficiency and how to avoid iron deficiency
in the third trimester of pregnancy 34
The importance of iron sufficiency 34
Great sources for iron 36

Taking iron supplements 37
Tips for getting as much iron as possible from foods you eat 38
Quiz: facts about nutrition during pregnancy 39
Chapter 5: 5 healthy recipes as suggestions for pregnant women 43
Recipe 1. Brocco mac and cheese (dinner) 43
Recipe 2. Pumpkin spice parfait (breakfast) 45
Recipe 3. Taco salad (dinner) 47
Recipe 4. Peachy crunchy yogurt (snack) 49
Recipe 5. Blueberry almond smoothie 50
Conclusion 51

INTRODUCTION

During the nine months of pregnancy, it may be exciting time when you know you are creating a new life, but this time may also make you confused because you have to experience numerous physical and hormonal changes in your body. When you are pregnant, alongside the change of the size of your belly and your lifestyle you have to experience, your nutritional needs during this time also increase because you do not only eat for yourself but also for your baby. Therefore, the foods you eat become the main source of nourishment for your baby and the way you nourish your body during this time will affect both of you and your baby's development in uterus. Furthermore, you're eating habits during pregnancy also

NUTRITION DURING PREGNANCY

affect your baby's eating habits in later life. For such reasons, it is important to know what you should eat and avoid during this time.

However, not all of us are good at this topic. Knowing the importance of nutrition to the health of moms-to-be and the baby's development during pregnancy and to help pregnant women to be well-equipped with basic knowledge related to nutrition during pregnancy as well, this book included 6 chapters will be the useful information about essential nutrients and guides for healthy eating habits during pregnancy for moms-to-be to have. Hopefully, after reading this, you will know what moms-to-be should eat and not to eat during pregnancy and the small tips come in every chapter will be actually valuable for you. Furthermore, this book is also aimed to the all readers regardless of sex and age but interested in the topic will have a great resource to learn about nutrition during pregnancy.

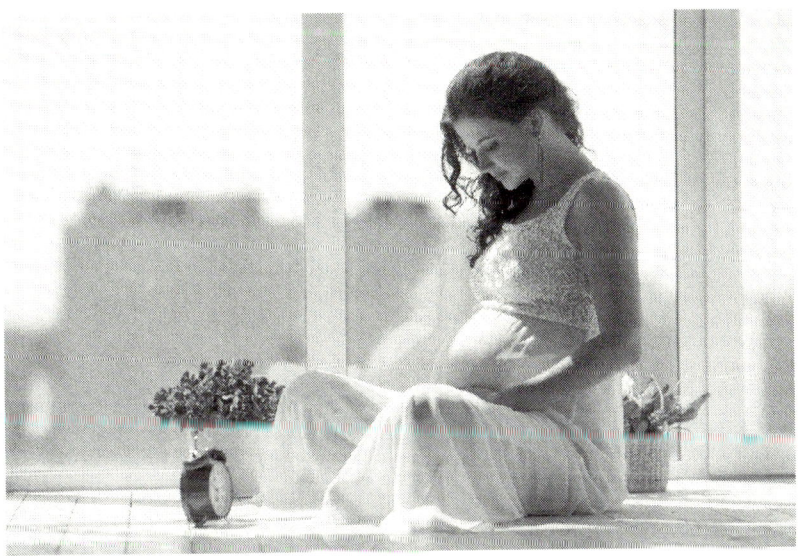

Chapter 1. 7 Golden Rules of Nutrition for Pregnant Women

Rule 1 – Don't Eat for Two

Many women think that pregnant women should eat more than they did before pregnancy because during this time they are eating for two persons but it turns out a misconception. You actually need an increasing amount of certain nutrients during pregnancy but it doesn't mean you have to eat double your portions or eat too much unless you want to end up with being overweight and cesarean delivery because your baby is too large. Furthermore, putting on too much weight during pregnancy can increase the risks of health problems including gestational diabetes. Bear in mind that the quality of foods you eat is better than the quantity of them, so focus on what nutrients contained in every food you eat instead of the quantity of them.

Rule 2 – Getting Enough Folic Acid

Folic Acid or folate is a vitamin B that plays an important role in the development of baby during pregnancy. In fact, folic acid helps to prevent certain malformations of the brain, skull and spine called neural tube defects (NTDs) including spina bifida and anencephaly and the sufficient intake of folic acid can reduce the chance of serious birth defects such as spina bifida by 50 % to 70 %.

In addition, birth defects often occur at very early stage of baby's development, often in the first four weeks of pregnancy when most women do not even realize they are pregnant, so it's important to have adequate folic acid intake when your baby's brain and spinal cord are developing. Furthermore, folic acid also helps to reduce your risk of preeclampsia as well as premature delivery. But how much does a woman need during pregnancy? The recommendation is that a pregnant woman needs 400 micrograms (mcg) a day and to reduce the risk for neural tube defects, so it would be ideal to take folic acid daily at least 3 months before you are planning on becoming pregnant and continue to take during your pregnancy.

Rule 3 – Getting Adequate Iron

You are advised to get 30 milligrams of iron per day for enough using of both you and your baby because during pregnancy your body needs an extra amount of iron to make more blood for your healthy baby's development. In addition, iron deficiency during pregnancy often makes you feel weak and tired. Most importantly severe iron deficiency can cause preterm delivery, low-birth-weight baby or even unborn death. Therefore, it's important to take considerations about adding iron-rich foods to your daily meals. If you are diagnosed with severe iron-deficiency, you could take iron supplements but you should do it under your doctor's supervision.

Rule 4 – Getting enough Zinc

Zinc plays an essential role in a great number of bodily activities including the construction of your baby's cells and forming DNA during pregnancy. In fact, Zinc is a necessary nutrient for cell division and tissue growth, supporting normal development as your baby grows. In addition, it also helps to support your immune system, maintain your sense of taste and smell and heal wounds. Although the deficiency of Zinc in human is rare, it also need to be paid attention to, particularly while you are pregnant because Zinc deficiency during pregnancy is linked to premature delivery and low-birth weight, so it is very important for women during pregnancy to get enough Zinc and a pregnant woman would need 11 milligrams of Zinc per day for the normal development of baby.

It may be not necessary to take Zinc supplements during pregnancy because there is a variety of Zinc-enriched foods that can give you enough Zinc intake such as meat, poultry, beans and nuts, etc. *Here are some foods that are high in Zinc for pregnant women:*

- Oyster: 15 mg per 1 cup
- Beef: (85 percent lean): 5.5 mg per 3 ounces.
- Spinach: 0.8 mg per 100 g.
- Cashews: 5.6mg per 100 g.
- Pumpkin seeds: 10.3 mg per 100 g.

Rule 5–Boosting Calcium Intake

Calcium is an essential nutrient to support your strong bones. When you are pregnant, you need about 1000 milligrams (mg) per day for the healthy development of your baby's bones and teeth, especially in the second and the third trimester of pregnancy when the baby's skeleton is developing strongly. Plus, if you experience calcium deficiency during pregnancy, your baby in uterus will take it from your bones for enough using, which often make you suffer from osteoporosis later in life. Therefore, for such importance of calcium, you should take a consideration on taking sufficient calcium for your baby's healthy development by eating calcium-rich foods daily. Milk and dairy products are great sources for calcium, for example, with 1 cup of plain skim-milk yogurt you eat, your body gets 488 mg of calcium and 8 ounces of skim milk will give you about 301 mg of calcium. You may be surprised that it is very easy to get enough the amount of calcium intake just by only drinking milk every day because 1000 mg of calcium is equivalent to three 8-ounce milk glasses. Therefore, just start your way for boosting calcium intake by drinking and eating at least 3 servings of dairy products as well as eating calcium-rich foods every day to ensure you won't experience calcium deficiency. In addition, don't forget to add to your daily meals with other calcium-rich foods like canned fishes because 3 ounces of canned pink salmon with bones and liquid can give you about 181 mg. However, to help your calcium absorption be better, here are some considerations that you should take.

- Foods that are rich in sodium inhibit the absorption of calcium, so you should reduce the consumption of processed foods and meats.
- Caffeine can slow calcium absorption, so it would be better to skip your favorite coffee in the mornings during pregnancy.
- Oxalates found in tea also slow the calcium's absorption, so if you are a fan of tea, just try to replace it with milk during pregnancy.
- Vitamin D promotes calcium absorption, so you can pair the calcium-rich foods with vitamin D-rich foods to have a better absorption.

Rule 6 – Focusing On Fiber

Fiber is an important part of healthy diet and it is more important when you are pregnant because during this time, your body often experiences constipation and digestive tract problems. Although these are the common problems that often occur during pregnancy, it may become bad to worse when constipation can lead to hemorrhoids. However, there is no use worrying about these problems because they can be easily minimized or eliminated by having enough fiber. How can you do that? Just learn these first. There are two types of fibers:

Insoluble fiber which does not dissolve in water can keep the digestive system work well. This type makes the pH balance of the intestines be kept under control as well as help to speed up the movement of waste material through the digestive system, so it can help you prevent constipation. Where can you get fiber on your diet? Fruits, vegetables, dried peas, beans and even whole grains are great sources for insoluble fiber.

Soluble fiber is partially dissolve in water can pair with fatty acids and keep you feeling full. In addition, it can help to regulate the sugar level in your blood as well as make your blood cholesterol at lower level. Where is this type of fiber found? It is contained in fruits, vegetables, oats, barley and dried peas, so add these foods to your meals for your adequate fiber intake.

Finally, getting at least 25 milligrams to 35 milligrams of fiber a day is a recommendation for a woman during pregnancy.

Rule 7 – Avoiding Harmful Foods and Drinks

Pregnant women should eat a variety of foods to ensure the sufficient nutrients and minerals to keep their body healthy and support the safe baby's development all nine months of pregnancy, but not all women are experts on what they should eat or avoid. Here are harmful foods women should keep away during pregnancy.

Unpasteurized dairy foods – Some foods like feta, goat cheese, Camembert and Brie are harmful to the health of baby inside the body because they are made from unpasteurized milk. These foods often contain listeria and bacteria which may lead to miscarriage and preterm delivery.

Hot dogs and luncheon meats including deli ham, turkey and salami – These foods are also prone to listeria which can change in your immune system during pregnancy and lead to your weaker defense against the infection than usual, so if you are in the mood for eating these types, you should reheat them before you eat to ensure all listeria and bacterium are completely killed.

Certain seafood and fish – Fish is known as a great source for omega-3 fatty acids that help baby's brain development. However, there are some kinds of fishes that pregnant women should avoid due to high levels of methyl-mercury which can interfere with the normal development of the growing child's brain and nervous system. They are shark, tilefish, swordfish and king mackerel.

Raw vegetable and sprouts – Raw vegetable and sprouts often contain bacteria no matter how carefully you wash them. Therefore, instead of eating them raw, you can cook them in different ways.

Alcohol drinks – Beers and wines aren't definitely good for our health if we consume them too much in the body, pregnant women are not exception. If a pregnant woman has alcohol drinks like wine, alcohol can pass from the mother's blood into the baby's blood, and then affect the growth of the baby's cells, brain and spinal cord cells. Furthermore, if the baby in uterus is exposed to alcohol, he will be smaller than other children of the same age in his later life after born.

Tea and coffee – Coffee may be your favorite drink in the mornings but here are two reasons that you should skip this kind of drink while you are pregnant.

Caffeine contained in coffee is a stimulant and a diuretic. Therefore, it can increase your blood pressure and heart rate, which is not good for your health. In addition, it causes the frequency of urination and leads to dehydration.

Caffeine can cross the placenta to your baby and inhibit the metabolism of your baby. In addition, caffeine is stimulant, so it can keep both you and your baby awake.

Chapter 2. Things to Consider in The First Trimester of Pregnancy

Dealing with Morning Sickness

Morning sickness is the common symptom that starts in early pregnancy and usually peaks at the ninth week of pregnancy. During this time, pregnant women often experience nausea or vomit which is caused by high levels of pregnancy hormones flooding your body. However, the term "morning sickness" often makes many people misled, not all of pregnant women feel sick in the mornings. On the contrary, nausea and vomiting can come at any time of the day, so the term doesn't accurately describe what most women experience. In addition, pregnancy-related nausea varies from woman to woman and not all of pregnant women actually vomit during morning sickness time. However, if you are experiencing vomit many times a day which leads to become dehydrated, along with feeling unusually fatigued and producing very little urine as well, you should ask your doctor for a check as soon as possible to know whether you suffer from hyperemesis gravidarum (HG) – a severe form of morning sickness because HG is different from normal morning sickness, it can affect you and your baby's health if it isn't treated. Furthermore, most pregnant women may concern about whether morning sickness affects the baby. The fact is there is no need to worry about morning sickness because it is a good sign to know that the placenta has developed well and your pregnancy hormones are working well to make sure that your baby gets enough what he needs from your body.

There are some factors that contribute to severe morning sickness in pregnancy including being deficient in certain nutrients such as vitamin B6 and magnesium, so you can ask your doctor to take vitamin B6 and magnesium supplements in order to help you go through morning sickness better. In addition, having a balance-diet with nutrient-rich foods is also advisable for pregnant women.

Here are some useful tips that may help ease your morning sickness:

Experiment with ginger – With no serious side effects, ginger has long been used to reduce the symptom of nausea and vomiting for pregnant women, so adding a thin slice of ginger to hot water or tea and drink your cup of ginger tea after meals can also stave off your nausea or you can also chew on crystallized ginger as your snack.

Eat a little – but more often – It would be better to divide your meals into six meals than three big meals a day as usual because when your stomach is empty, stomach acids have nothing to feast on, but when eating too much can overtax the digestive system and both of them can trigger nausea, so keeping your stomach a little bit full all day and all night is the best way to help ease your morning sickness.

Stay hydrated – It sounds unbelievable to many of us, but the more hydrated you are, the less nauseated you'll become, so try to drink eight glasses of water every day to let your body get enough liquid in.

Avoid unpleasant smells – While morning sickness is occurring, you are very sensitive to certain smells. The smell of food your husband is cooking in the kitchen also make you dash for the toilet, so just stay away from anything can cause your nausea and vomiting.

Sniff lemon – Although you may have an aversion to certain smells during the morning sickness time, but sniffing something sour like lemon also helps sometimes. Drinking lemonade or orange juice is also worth a try.

Lie down and take a rest from work – Morning sickness is difficult to ignore, but when your nausea is coming, it would better to take a rest from work and lie down, take a few deep breaths, close your eyes and trying to take a nap.

Certain Nutrient-deficiency Is Linked to Miscarriage

Most early miscarriages in early pregnancy are caused by genetic abnormalities. However, being deficient in certain nutrients can also contribute to higher risks for miscarriage. As a few studies have shown that pregnant women who are lower at folic acid level put themselves at higher risk for early miscarriage, so alongside reducing their unborn baby's risk of neural tube defects, taking enough folic acid also help to prevent miscarriage. That's why you're advised to have 400 mcg of folic acid intake every day but instead of taking folic acid supplements you can meet your folic acid need just by eating folic acid-rich foods.

Foods Are High in Folic Acid

1. Dark Leafy Green

If you are looking for natural ways to obtain your folic acid, don't forget these leafy greens because they are packed with a lot of nutrients including folic acid.

- Spinach — 263 mcg of folate (65% DV) per 1 cup
- Collard Greens — 177 mcg of folate (44% DV) per 1 cup
- Turnip Greens — 170 mcg of folate (42% DV) per 1 cup
- Mustard Greens — 103 mcg of folate (26% DV) per 1 cup
- Romaine Lettuce — 76 mcg of folate (19% DV) per 1 cup

2. Bean, Peas and Lentils

All beans, peas and lentils are rich in folic acid, so you will never worry about lack of your folic acid intake if you are just a fan of one certain type of beans.

- Lentils — 358 mcg of folate (90% DV) per 1 cup
- Black Beans — 256 mcg of folate (64% DV) per 1 cup
- Kidney Beans — 229 mcg of folate (57% DV) per 1 cup

- Green Peas — 101 mcg of folate (25% DV) per 1 cup
- Green Beans — 42 mcg of folate (10% DV) per 1 cup

3. Avocados

Being the favorite fruit of many people, avocado is high in folic acid with 90 mcg of folate contained in 1 cup of avocado which account for approximately 22% of your daily need. This tropical fruit becomes an excellent one for making salads, smoothies or eat raw.

4. Cauliflower and broccoli

These two vegetables have long been known as great sources for folic acid. Eating just one cup of cauliflower will give you about 55 mcg of folate, which accounts for approximately 14% of your recommended daily value and 1 cup broccoli contain about 104 mcg of folate which is equivalent to ¼ of your daily need.

5. Seeds and Nuts

Seeds and nuts are also good choices for boosting your folate intake, so add one of these types of seeds and nuts more often to your recipes.

- Sunflower Seeds — 82 mcg of folate (21% DV) per ¼ cup
- Peanuts — 88 mcg of folate (22%) per ¼ cup
- Almonds — 46 mcg of folate (12% DV) per 1 cup

Chapter 3. Nutritional Requirements in The Second Trimester of Pregnancy

Protein

Each nutrient plays a particular role in the body and so protein is. Protein helps the metabolism in the body better and keeps you feel full longer. Most importantly, the building blocks of your body's cells and of your baby's body are formed by the amino acids found in protein. In addition, proteins help to repair muscle tissue and red blood cells. They carry nutrients and oxygen to cells and prevent blood clotting as well, particularly those in the uterus and placenta. Therefore, during pregnancy, protein becomes more important for baby's development, especially in the second and the third trimester of pregnancy when your baby's brain will be developing faster.

The recommended daily need for protein per day varies from person to person. It is based on the weight of each individual and a recommendation for a safe protein intake is about 0.8 grams of protein per kilogram of body weight. For instance, a regular woman of 64 kg who is engaged in moderate physical activities would need 51 grams of protein. When being pregnant, she will need about 76 grams of protein per day.

All foods such as meat, seafood, beans, and seeds are packed with protein, but every type of them will have different amount in one serving, so knowing what amount constitutes one serving helps you count the proper requirement for protein you need. *Here is what you need to know:*

Dairy products:

- 1 cup of cottage cheese (low-fat): 24 g
- 8 ounces of yogurt (low-fat): around 10 g
- 1 ounce of Parmesan cheese: 11 g
- 1 cup of low-fat milk: 8 g
- 1 ounce of cheddar cheese: 7 g

Meat, poultry and fish:

- 1/2 chicken breast without skin: 27 g
- 3 ounces of sockeye salmon and trout (grilled): 23 g
- 1 ounces of lean beef (broiled): 7g

Beans, nuts, legumes:

- 1 cup of raw tofu firm: 40 g
- 1 cup of lentils: 18 g
- 1 cup of canned black beans: 15 g
- 1 cup of canned kidney beans: 13 g
- 1 tablespoons of smooth peanut butter: 4 g
- 1 cup of light plain soymilk: 6 g

Omega-3 fatty Acids

You are often advised to take enough omega-3 fatty acids due to the plenty benefits of omega3-fatty acids including preventing heart disease, especially, women who are pregnant need an extra amount of omega-3 fatty acids to ensure the healthy development of the baby of the mother.

There are three types of omega-3 fatty acids including ALA, EPA and DHA. Among them EPA (eicosapentaenoic acid) and DHA (docosahexaenoic acid) are two most beneficial to pregnant women. Although these two types of omega3-fatty acids can work together, each type has its own unique benefits. EPA helps to support the heart, immune system and inflammatory response whereas DHA is important for your baby's visual and neurological development.

Along with other benefits that omega3-fatty acids bring to your health regardless of who you are, omega-3 fatty acids have more positive effects while you are pregnant, you will need an increase amount of EPA and DHA to prevent pre-term delivery, lower the risk of preeclampsia and avoid low birth weight. Plus, omega3-fatty acid deficiency is also associated with the mother's risk for depression. However, where can you get omega3-fatty acids? Fish has long been known as a great source for omega3-fatty acids, but the problem is not all fishes are safe to pregnant women because many of them are high in mercury which can affect the baby's growing brain and nervous system. This is why many women struggle with whether they should eat fishes during pregnancy or not, and many of these women often end up with skipping fishes in their meals as a way to stay safe for their baby. However, this is necessary to keep fishes away from your meals because fishes are not only low in saturated fat but also great sources for protein, vitamin D, and other nutrients that are essential for a developing baby and a healthy pregnancy, so how eat fishes to avoid mercury but still get omega3-fatty acids and other nutrients? *Here comes with questions and answers as guides:*

1. Question: Which fishes are often high in mercury?

    Answer: They are shark, swordfish, king mackerel, and tilefish.

2. Question: How much fish should a pregnant woman eat per day?

    Answer: Eating 8 to 12 ounces of fish low in mercury per week which is equivalent to about 2 to 3 servings of fish per week as the recommendation of FDA.

3. Question: What happens if a pregnant woman eats fishes that are high in mercury?

Answer: It is based on how much she has eaten, but one serving of such a fish wouldn't put her on a risk.

4. Question: What about fishes that are caught in local water?
   Answer: The safety of them depends on the water of your lake, river and coastal area. If it is caught in near a contaminated region, it is better to avoid.

5. Question: Is it safe to eat sushi during pregnancy?
   Answer: Sushi can be made with safe fishes like salmon but it is still better to stay away from sushi and other dishes made with raw fish because raw fishes often contain parasites, harmful viruses and bacteria which are not good for both health of the mother and baby.

However, if you are not a fan of fishes where else can you get omega3-fatty acids as replacements? You can take omega3-fatty acid supplements, but please ask your doctor for advices to know exactly how much safe dose of omega3-fatty acids you should really need. Furthermore, there are still great sources for omega3-fatty acids you can obtain through your diet including eggs, liver, milk, soy beverages and others omega3-fatty acids come in plant foods like walnuts and flaxseeds.

Chapter 4. Staying Healthy and Safe in the Last Trimester of Pregnancy

How to Manage Healthy Weight in The Last Trimester of Pregnancy

Being overweight during pregnancy can lead to complications for both of you and your baby. The more overweight you are, the more likely that you will put yourself high risks of health problems including obesity, gestational diabetes, high blood pressure and cesarean delivery. But how do you know you are overweight? If your body mass index (BMI) before you are pregnant is between 25.0 and 29.9, this means you are overweight. If your BMI reaches to 30.0 and above, it is worse because you are putting yourself at risks for health problems including diabetes linked to being obese. Here are guides to calculate your BMI and an amount of healthy weight you should gain in the third trimester of pregnancy.

Formula: Weight (kg) / [height (m)]^2 = result (BMI).

Example: Weight = 68 kg and Height = 165 cm (1.65m)

Calculation: 68/ (1.65)^2 = 24, 98

And here is the table that shows how the BMI is associated with your weights.

NUTRITION DURING PREGNANCY

BMI	Weight Status	Recommended range of total weight (pounds)	Recommended rates of weight gain in the third trimester (pounds) (means range lb/week)
Below 18.5	Under weight	28 - 40	1 (1 -1.3)
18.5 – 24.9	Healthy weight	25 - 35	1 (0.8 – 1)
25.0 – 29.9	Overweight	15 - 25	0.6 (0.5 – 0.7)
30.0 and above	Obese	11 - 20	0.5 (0.4 – 0.6)

Explanation: One pound = 0.454 kg

For example: If a woman weighs 68 kg and has a height of 1.65m before she is pregnant, she will get her BMI of 24,98. This means she has a normal or healthy weight, so when she is pregnant she will need to gain between 25 – 35 pounds which are equivalent to 6 kg to 15 kg to make sure the healthy development of the baby. Are you wondering how your body uses 35 pounds of weight? Here are the numbers in the details for 35 pounds of weight you gain.

- Placenta: 2 to 3 pounds
- Amniotic fluid: 2 to 3 pounds
- Breast tissue: 2 to 3 pounds
- Uterus growth: 2 to 5 pounds
- Blood supply: 4 pounds
- Baby: 8 pounds
- Fat stores: 5 to 9 pounds

How Many Calories Do You Need During Pregnancy?

Gaining weight during pregnancy is encouraged for women, but gaining too much weight can cause problems that are harmful to both of you and your baby. In fact, the amount of calorie intake is closely related to gaining weight. That's why to manage your weight, you have to regular your calorie intake, but have you already known the right amount of calories that a pregnant woman really needs to get? If you are pregnant, you are recommended to get about 1,800 calories per day in the first trimester and 2,200 calories per day in the second trimester. In the last trimester, your body would need an extra of calories, about 200 calories of extra amount per day which equals to 2400 calories per day to support the growing baby. However, if you are gaining two pounds per week in the third trimester of pregnancy, it means you are highly facing cesarean deliver because of your too-large baby. It would be quite late to regulate your weight if you are near the due date, so creating a healthy eating habit should be done as early as possible if you want to avoid experiencing a cesarean delivery and get back into shape as soon as possible after birth.

NUTRITION DURING PREGNANCY

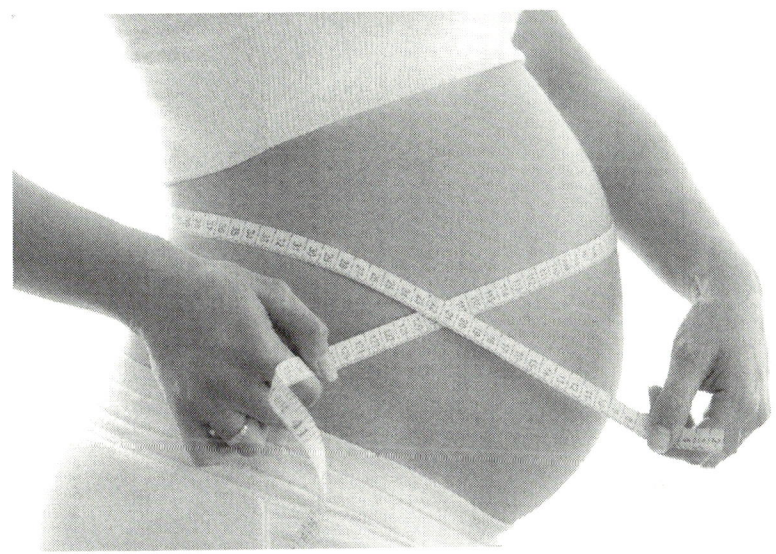

Tips to Manage Your Weight:

1. Eat moderately and often

It is better to have 4 – 6 meals with a small portion in each instead of 3 big meals. The fact is after eating your body needs time to burn the calories and it takes about 3 hours for fully digestion a meal. When you eat a big meal at once time, the calories you burn are less than the calories you consume and the excess calories will be stored as fat, which causes overweight. However, by eating smaller meals and eating often, you can prevent this and your body doesn't need to store calories as fat for later use, so you will be provided the usual energy and stable sugar blood level.

2. Drink Enough Water

You're recommended to drink 8 glasses of water to avoid dehydration during pregnancy. Most importantly you need to drink enough water to help your digestive system speed up, avoid constipation and prevent uncomfortable floating. In addition, water also helps you feel longer full, which really means when you want to avoid excess calories from foods.

3. Choosing Nonfat Dairy Products and Skimmed Milk

Dairy products are great sources for protein and calcium but are also high in calories, fat and cholesterol, which are not good for your health, so you can replace them with nonfat dairy products and skimmed milk to limit your calories and cholesterol intake.

4. Reducing Junk Foods

Junk foods are often packed with a lot of sugar and fat which make you put on weight quickly but your body doesn't get enough the amount of calories you need, so keep them away or reduce the amount of junk food you eat daily as a way for healthy eating habit during pregnancy.

5. Eliminating sugar and sweetened drinks

Sweetened drinks are full of sugar which is linked to an increase of risk of insulin resistance and cause overweight. A 12-ounce can of sugary soda which is equal to 340 ml contains 38 grams of carbs which can provide you half of calories from them, so instead of soft drinks juice, fruits are healthier.

6. Don't Skip Your Breakfast

Many people think that skipping breakfast may help them lose weight, but this isn't good, particularly pregnant women. Skipping breakfast may make your morning sickness become worse due to energy deficiency and ravenous hunger.

7. Eating more fruits and vegetables

Fruits and vegetables are packed with a lot of vitamins such as vitamin A, C, E, K and they not also contain natural sugar which is healthier to your body but are also high in fiber to help you have a better digestion. Therefore, for such benefits, why don't you add more fruits and vegetables to the list of what you should eat during pregnancy?

The Importance of Iron Sufficiency and How to Avoid Iron Deficiency in The Third Trimester of Pregnancy

The Importance of Iron Sufficiency

As being mentioned in the rule 2 of chapter 1, iron plays an important role for the mother and the baby. Particularly in the third trimester of pregnancy, most women experience iron deficiency, that's why it is needed to have a further discussion about the importance of sufficient iron in the body during nine months of pregnancy.

Iron is a component of hemoglobin - a protein found in red blood cells that carries oxygen around the body. During pregnancy, your body needs more iron to make extra blood for you and your baby, especially in the third trimester of pregnancy. Therefore, to support the healthy growth of your baby, the amount of blood in your body must increase up to 50% and you may need about twice the amount of iron as you did before, often about 30 milligrams per day.

If your body don't have enough iron to make the hemoglobin for your need you become anemic. When iron-deficiency anemia occurs in early or mid-pregnancy, it may lead to preterm delivery, low-birth-weight baby or even unborn death, so that's why it is very important to get adequate iron during pregnancy. However, how do you know whether you are deficient in iron or not? *Here are signs:*

Feeling Exhausted – When iron level is low in your body, there is less oxygen to reach your tissues, so your body will lack the energy it needs. That's why you will feel tired, week and even get out of breath easily when doing things like going up stairs, plus sometimes you will feel irritable, dizzy or difficult to focus on.

Pale-looking skin – Because hemoglobin gives your blood its red color and makes your skin its rosy hue, so if your skin looks pale and the inside of your bottom eyelids are less red than usual, think of iron deficiency immediately!

Loosing hair – A lot of women experience loosing hair during pregnancy and most of losing hair cases of pregnant women are linked to iron-deficiency. Plus, the loosing hair is considered severe when there are over one hundred of hair losses per day.

Craving for non-food substances – During pregnancy, it is common to see women crave for certain foods or even have an aversion to foods they liked before pregnancy. But if you are tending to crave for non-foods substances like clay, dirt and ice, you are having signs of iron-deficiency and this condition is also known as pica.

Great Sources for Iron

Getting enough iron is significantly important to reduce risks of preterm delivery, low birth weight and newborn death for women. Therefore, there is no way better than getting iron naturally by eating a variety of iron-rich foods every day. But where are great sources for iron? All foods from both of animals and plants are rich in iron. However, heme iron found in only animal foods is easier to absorb than non-heme iron found in iron-fortified foods, supplements and foods from all kinds.

Iron-rich foods from animals:

- Lean beef: 3.2 mg of iron per 3 ounces
- Lean beef tenderloin: 1.0 mg of iron per 1 ounce
- Roast turkey: 2.0 mg iron of per 3 ounces
- Roast turkey breast: 1.4 mg of iron per 3 ounces
- Roast chicken: 1.1 mg of iron per 3 ounces
- Roast chicken breast: 1.1 mg of iron per 3 ounces
- Pork loin: 0.8 mg of iron per 3 ounces

Iron-rich foods from plants:

- Lentils (cooked): 6.6 mg of iron per 1 cup
- Kidney beans (cooked): 5.2 mg of iron per 1 cup

- Chickpeas: 4.8 mg of iron per 1 cup
- Lima beans: 4.5 mg of iron per 1 cup
- Pumpkin seeds (roasted): 4.2 mg of iron per 1 ounce
- Boiled spinach: 6.4 mg of iron per 1 cup
- Prune juice: 3.0 mg of iron per 1 cup
- Raisin: 30 mg of iron per 1 cup

Note: It is advisable to not eat liver, liver products including liver sausage and pate although these are top foods that are high in iron because liver is often high in vitamin A which may be harmful to your unborn baby.

Taking Iron Supplements

Poor nutrients in your daily meals may not give your body adequate iron you need during pregnancy, it's time to take iron supplements but it is better to ask your doctor to have a right guide on how much dose you really need because unlike other nutrients, an excess iron level in your body can lead to health problems including constipation, nausea, diarrhea and tummy upsets. If you are not anemia, you are recommended to take 30 mg of iron.

Tips for Getting as Much Iron as Possible from Foods You Eat

- It is advisable to avoid drinking coffee, tea and alcohol near the time you take an iron supplement or at the same time you're having your meals because these drinks may inhibit the iron absorption.
- Calcium isn't also good when it is paired with iron because calcium will reduce the iron absorption, so if you have to take calcium supplements, don't take calcium supplements and iron supplements at the same time.
- Vitamin C can help to promote the iron absorption up to six times, so it is best to pair two of them together. You can have a glass of orange juice after meals to help your body get enough vitamin C intake as well as increase your iron absorption.

NUTRITION DURING PREGNANCY

To check your knowledge on nutrition during pregnancy, here is a quiz for you to do, just circle your answer and check them after finishing:

Quiz: Facts about nutrition during pregnancy

1. Morning sickness only occurs in the mornings?
    a. True
    b. False
2. Ginger may help ease your morning sickness?
    a. True
    b. False
3. Sushi is completely safe for pregnant women?
    a. True
    b. False
4. How much fish should a woman eat during pregnancy?
    a. No more than 3 ounces per week
    b. 5 ounces per week
    c. 5 - 7 ounces per week
    d. 8 - 12 ounces per week
5. When you should start taking folic acid supplements?
    a. As soon as you are pregnant
    b. When you are planning on getting pregnant
    c. Even when you are not trying to get pregnant
    d. When you are diagnosed with folic acid deficiency
6. Which craving could be a sign of iron deficiency?
    a. Carrot
    b. Pizza

c. Coffee

d. Ice

7. Which of the following cheeses is not good for pregnant women?

    a. Gouda

    b. Mozzarella

    c. Feta

    d. Romano

8. If you eat a lot of avocados during pregnancy, your baby is likely to enjoy avocado, too.

    a. True

    b. False

9. Which fish is high in mercury?

    a. Salmon

    b. Shellfish

    c. Tilefish

    d. Catfish

10. Hot dogs and sausages are still alright for pregnant women to eat if they are reheated?

    a. True

    b. False

11. Non-heme iron is easier to absorb than heme-iron?

    a. True

    b. False

12. Non-heme iron is found in plant foods?

    a. True

b. False
13. An excess iron level in the body can cause constipation?
    a. True
    b. False
14. Liver is high in Iron?
    a. True
    b. False
15. Pregnant women are advisable to avoid liver due to being high in?
    a. Vitamin D
    b. Iron
    c. Vitamin C
    d. Vitamin A
16. Vitamin C can inhibit iron absorption?
    a. True
    b. False
17. Calcium can help to increase the iron absorption?
    a. True
    b. False
18. Which nutrient plays a crucial role in the construction of your baby's cells and DNA during pregnancy?
    a. Iron
    b. Calcium
    c. Protein
    d. Zinc
19. Which vitamin can promote the calcium absorption?

a. Vitamin A
b. Vitamin B
c. Vitamin C
d. Vitamin D

20. You're considered to have a healthy weight, when your BMI is?
a. 20
b. 24
c. 32
d. 35

Your correct answers:

Question	1	2	3	4	5	6	7	8	9	10
Answer	b	a	b	d	c	d	c	a	c	a
Question	11	12	13	14	15	16	17	18	19	20
Answer	b	a	a	a	d	b	b	d	d	b

Chapter 5. 5 Healthy Recipes as Suggestions for Pregnant Women

Recipe 1. Brocco Mac and Cheese (dinner)

Ingredients:

- Organic 1% milk – 2 cups
- Nonfat dry milk powder – 1 teaspoon
- Unsalted butter – 1 teaspoon
- All-purpose flour – 2 teaspoons
- Frozen chopped broccoli, thawed – 10 ounces
- Whole-wheat macaroni, cooked – 8 ounces
- Organic shredded cheddar cheese – 6 ounces
- Grated Parmesan cheese – 1 teaspoon
- Salt – ¼ teaspoon
- Freshly ground black pepper – ¼ teaspoon
- Dry breadcrumbs – ¼ cup

Instructions:

1. Preheat your oven to 350 degrees. Then spray your dish thinly with cooking oil and set aside.
2. Mix milk and milk powder well together in a bowl.

3. Using a saucepan to melt the butter at medium heat, then whisk in the flour. Cook, stirring constantly for two minutes.
4. Gradually add the milk to the mixture, whisk it well, then cook for about 5 minutes until mixture thickens and remove from heat.
5. Add the cheddar cheese, salt, and pepper to the warm milk mixture. Stir it well until the cheese melts. Mix it with the broccoli and cooked macaroni in a prepared baking dish, sprinkle the breadcrumbs and Parmesan on top, and then put it in the oven.
6. Bake it for about 30 minutes until it turns golden on top, then it is ready for serve.

Nutrient totals:

Calories – 276; Fat – 13 g; Cholesterol – 41 g; Protein – 16 g; Carbohydrate – 28 g; Sugars – 6 g; Fiber – 6 g; Iron – 1 mg; Sodium – 383 mg; Calcium – 360 mg; Folate – 37 mcg; Beta-Carotene – 290 mcg.

Recipe 2. Pumpkin Spice Parfait (breakfast)

Ingredients:

- Canned pumpkin puree – 1/3 cup
- Pumpkin pie spice – ¼ teaspoon
- Maple syrup – 2 teaspoons
- Nonfat plain yogurt – 1 cup
- Granola – 4 tablespoons
- Raisin – 2 tablespoons
- Chopped cashew – 4 teaspoons

Instructions:

1. Firstly, you add canned pumpkin puree, pumpkin pie spice, maple syrup and nonfat plain yogurt together, and mix them well.
2. Secondly, you divide the mixture you have mixed above into two equal portions, then put half amount of the mixture of pumpkin and yogurt into a glass, then add half amount of granola (2 tablespoons), half amount of raisins (1 tablespoon) and half amount chopped cashews (1 tablespoon) on the top.
3. Thirdly, repeat the second step with the same amount of all ingredients.
4. Finally, it is ready to serve.

Nutrients totals:

Calories – 455.4 g; protein – 20.7 g; Carbohydrates– 68g; Fiber – 6.357 g; fat – 13.0 g; Saturated fat - 2.824 g; Cholesterol – 4.41 mg; Calcium – 552.2 mg; Iron – 3.726 mg; Sodium – 199.6 mg; Folate – 71.0 mcg.

Recipe 3. Taco salad (dinner)

Ingredients: 4 servings

- Lean ground sirloin – 1 pound
- Cayenne pepper – ½ teaspoon
- Ground cumin – ½ teaspoon
- ½ cup plus 3 tbsp salsa, divided (hotness of your choice)
- Canned black beans, rinsed and drained – 15 ounces
- Light sour cream – 2 teaspoons
- Chopped romaine (about 1 head) – 8 cups
- Avocado – 1 and diced
- Chopped tomato - 1
- Fresh cilantro, for garnish – 2 teaspoons

Constructions:

1. Defrost the meat and chop it.
2. Add the chopped meat to a large pan and cook over medium heat, stir it with a spatula. Add the cayenne and cumin and cook 6 to 7 minutes. Remove from heat, and drain off the juices.
3. Add ½ cup salsa and the beans into the meat and stir the mix well, then return to medium heat. Cook about 2 minutes, then season with additional cayenne, salt, and pepper, if desired.
4. Meanwhile, add 3 tablespoons salsa to the sour cream in a small bowl, then mix it well together and set aside.
5. In a serving bowl, put lettuce equally, top with the meat mixture, chopped tomato, and diced avocados. Drizzle with the dressing garnish with cilantro, and serve.

Nutrient totals:

Calories – 340 g; Fat – 13 g (Sat 4 g, Mono 7 g, Poly 2 g); Cholesterol – 63 mg; Protein – 30 g; Carbohydrate – 28 g; Fiber – 8 g; Iron – 5 mg; Sodium – 384 mg; Calcium – 122 mg; Folate – 196 mg; Vitamin B12 – 2.4 mcg; Potassium – 564 mg; Zinc – 5 mg.

Recipe 4. Peachy Crunchy Yogurt (snack)

Ingredients:

- Non-fat yogurt – 6 ounces
- Peach - 1
- Flaxseeds – 2 teaspoons
- Granola – 1 teaspoon

Instructions:

This may be the easiest recipe to make you've ever done, because all you need to do is mix 6 ounces of non fat peach yogurt with 2 teaspoons of flaxseeds, 1 teaspoon granola and peach slices together and stir well, then serve.

Nutrient totals:

Calories - 198.7 g; Protein – 15.7 g; Carbohydrate – 25.2 g; Dietary Fiber – 2.002 g; Total Sugars – 19.1 g; Total Fat – 3. 854 g; Saturated Fat – 503 g; Total Omega-3 FA – 1.065 g; Calcium – 216.2 g; Iron – 543 g; Sodium – 67.1 mg; Vitamin C – 1.298 mg; Folate – 9.679 mg.

Recipe 5. Blueberry Almond Smoothie

Ingredients:

- Blueberry – ¾ cup
- Almond butter – 2 teaspoons
- Honey – 1 teaspoon
- Unsweetened soy milk/ yogurt – ¾ cup (you can use yogurt if you are not a fan of soy milk).

Instructions:

1. Add blueberries, 2 teaspoons almond butter, 1 teaspoon honey, and 3/4 cup unsweetened soy milk or yogurt together in your blender and press the button.
2. Pour the smoothie in a glass and ready to serve.

Nutrient totals:

Calories – 202.5 g; Protein – 6.787 g; Carbohydrate – 25.6 g; Dietary Fiber – 5.758 g; Total Sugars – 6.495 g; Total Fat – 9.487 g; Saturated Fat – 1.004 g; Total Omega-3 FA – 0.45 g; Calcium – 271.2 g; Iron – 1.835 g; Sodium – 68.4 g; Vitamin C – 1.895 g; Folate – 25.3 mcg.

Conclusion

You have to experience numerous both physically and emotionally challenges during nine months of pregnancy, which often alters your lifestyle. Each trimester you have to experience certain changes in your body, so the nutritional need is. Certain nutrient plays a particular role in each stage of development of your baby as well as your need for nutrients alters as your baby grows trimester by trimester. In fact, you are expected to get sufficient in all kinds of nutrients and minerals but not excess to support your baby's growth healthily and safely. Therefore, you seem to be more careful to not to do the wrong things because you are now living and eating for two. That's why knowing which rule in eating habits is good for you and your baby will help you minimize the chances of developing birth defects. In addition, being knowledgeable about changes which are waiting for you in each of trimester will help you deal with your condition better.

Knowing the nutritional need for each trimester of pregnancy is very important because nutritional requirements for each trimester is different and certain nutrient deficiency or excess can lead to health problems of the mother and the baby. Therefore, understanding what to expect for each trimester of pregnancy will help women to cope with those challenges better and these pieces of information are considered as golden rules to stay healthy, fit and comfortable during pregnancy. In addition, with practical guides to deal with health problems occurring in each trimester will be useful for pregnant women. Furthermore, the more knowledgeable the more confident you are when becoming a mom.

ABOUT THE AUTHOR

Hi, everybody! My name is Melanie and 28 years old. As a regular woman, I love the normal things like other regular people like. I love music, shopping, travelling, cooking and eating. As an eating lover luckily I'm not a picky eater. I can eat mostly everything and I must confess that I'm a big fan of coffee and my breakfast is always paired with a cup of coffee. To me food doesn't the thing that keep us survived it also has its own story which can be associated with the culture of where it is come from or the way it was invented or how it attects to health, so each new food I try to cook or eat makes me fascinated to learn the stories behind.

There are a few things that I would consider my first priority in life. They are my family, friends and career, so everything I do in life would be around these. I also witnessed the death of my uncle after having a long battle against his diabetes. Before that he had had to follow a strict diet and had to ignore a lot of great foods he liked because they are high in sugar, which sometimes bothered him a lot. I also have an aunt who isn't allowed to drink coffee and soya products by doctors due to having been diagnosed with hyperthyroidism. Therefore I understand that health is the key for everything. I mean that we can't enjoy all excitements in life without health, so everything can give me healthier is worth learning and trying, so food is a part of them.

And for those reasons my two books were written. Yeap, that's right! My two books are born with an ambition to remind everybody to pay more attention to what we eat, particularly in these two books, I give my priority to the health of women who are pregnant – the most beautiful time in life but also the vulnerable time they have to experience. Hope that with my two books I somewhat help the readers have not only basic knowledge about the importance of nutrition during pregnancy but also have great meals to eat in order to survive and to eat to be healthier.

Made in the USA
Lexington, KY
14 March 2019